THE REAL CAUSE OF PAIN AND SICKNESS

And What You Can Do About It

Andrew Cort, DC
53 Rock City Road
Woodstock, NY 12498
(845) 750-9652

For Marjorie

I would like to thank and acknowledge my debt to the many authors, teachers, healers, and thinkers who are mentioned in this book, and many who are not. I would especially like to thank my good friend and colleague Maryanne DiPalma Buchele for many excellent suggestions regarding content as well as her indispensable editing advice. Also thanks to Judi Boruta for the cover photo.

Contents

1. WHAT IS THE *REAL* CAUSE OF PAIN AND SICKNESS?

Fundamentally, we can say that ***stress and tension*** cause the body to develop pain and illness. It's a bit more complicated than this, there are more pieces to the puzzle, and *we will consider them all*. But we can safely begin by whittling things down to essentials and starting here.

Stress and tension, of course, can be caused by *many different factors*: perhaps most importantly, though not exclusively, by painful ***emotions***:

For example:

If you have little or no time for relaxation, fun, and playfulness, perhaps because of the need to work long, exhausting hours in order to survive and care for loved ones, or perhaps because you are so focused on a need for financial achievement that you don't give yourself time to slow down, *your body will become tense.*

If you are enduring a life of difficult, perhaps even abusive, family dynamics, or if you are constantly trying to please and accommodate others at the cost of your own hopes and desires, *your body will become tense.*

If you are constantly living with conflict, physical danger, impossible demands, or are being constantly exposed to hatred, anger or violence, *your body will become tense.*

If you are struggling with money issues (as so many folks are), or can't find work, and are panicking or feeling ashamed or inadequate (worried perhaps that you can't be a good parent or spouse because you are always lacking money), *your body will become tense.*

If you have *already* fallen ill, are suffering with pain, have been told "it's all in your head" or "nothing can be done", or you fear that you may never be well again, your *body will become **even more** tense.*

If you cope with life's difficulties by "putting them out of your head" and telling yourself that you are carefree and easygoing, *the body will know better and the body will become tense.* In fact, John Sarno, M.D., in his little book *Mind Over Back Pain*, noted that "This is a foolproof formula for generating tension. Putting things out of one's mind doesn't get rid of them; it simply relegates them to the unconscious, where they are free to create anxiety undisturbed. This hidden tension then manifests itself in a physical disorder....."[*]

Sarno goes on to suggest that our unpleasant emotions lead to physical illness and pain because this is a safe way to distract us from unacceptable feelings: so *to protect ourselves* from too much negative emotion, we channel the tension elsewhere, i.e., into the body. Anyway, insurance companies are more likely to cover *physical* ailments, and there is far less stigma.

~

There are **many other sources of stress and tension** besides these emotions: physical trauma; polluted air, food, or water; lack of sleep; too much or too little exercise; poor nutrition; dental problems; hunger; grief and a sense of emptiness or loss; feeling lonely and unloved; drugs or other addictions; feeling oppressed by all the sadness in the world; feeling overly vulnerable or bullied; PTSD (post-traumatic stress disorder. experienced by many war veterans, catastrophe survivors, abused individuals, and others); feeling unsafe or oppressed; an onslaught of germs/pathogens; genetic issues; taking on the negative energies of other people; perhaps even the effects of karma or past lives.

So we see that the causes of pain and illness can actually be quite varied and complex. After all, we are unique multifaceted individuals, endlessly changing, endlessly growing: we are *not* merely identical physical machines that can be periodically repaired or upgraded with synthetic chemicals. **We are physical, emotional, psychological, social, and spiritual beings**. To be truly healthy, *all* these aspects of our existence must be functioning well, and in a balanced, harmonious relationship with each other and with the outer world.

This human complexity explains why there are many different kinds of health practitioners, each concerned with only one or a few of these factors, and trained to work only with those particular factors. Sadly, the resulting fragmentation of these efforts (exacerbated by a lack of respect and communication among the professions) is why many chronically ill people find themselves going from one practitioner to another, trying first this therapy and then that one, often getting nowhere, and typically becoming *even more stressed.*

The marketplace is filled with books and experts espousing diverse and contradictory information on how to heal and be healthy. To help sort this all out, *rather than adding* to the confusion I'm going to *draw all this information together* into *a simple unified theory of disease and healing.*

---

[*] Sarno, John M.D., *Mind Over Back Pain,* Berkley Books, NY, 1986, p. 53

In other words, I am going to suggest an inclusive, coherent, **definition of 'Holistic'** that can *help you make effective decisions*.

In addition to bringing some clarity to the discussion, I hope this will challenge much of the ingrained, orthodox *way of thinking* about health and disease that sees all illness as an invading entity that must be destroyed.* I say this because when health care is concerned only with combatting disease and symptoms, this attitude – in addition to being an unnecessarily violent way of approaching life and health – allows us to indulge in the dangerous illusion that we can keep doing everything wrong (to ourselves, to each other, and to the planet) and we will somehow "get away with it" (for instance, since scientists will eventually rid us of heart disease, we can keep eating badly). **But changing nothing about oneself, while waiting for a magical cure, is a terrible mistake.**

~

This unifying idea is based on the ancient concept that everything which comes into existence has three inherent 'forces' or qualities:

An "**Active**" force

A "**Receptive**" force, and

A "**Conciliating**" force.

This simply means that for anything to occur:

(1) something must *'act'*, i.e., *do something* (the active force),

(2) something must *'receive'* the action (the receptive force), and then,

(3) something must *mediate between them* and determine the precise relationship that eventuates (the conciliating force).

Perhaps the simplest way of seeing this idea at work is in chemistry. In a basic chemical experiment, a chemical, called a re-agent, is placed in a test tube (this represents the receptive force waiting to be acted upon). Another chemical is then added, to act upon the first one (this is called the agent, representing the active force). But nothing happens until a third force, a 'catalyst', is added, that arouses and guides the interaction

---

* The worst kind of medicine is *descriptive only:* it 'names' your disease and treats the name, but it is not even interested in *why* these symptoms are happening, or why they are happening to *you.*

3

between the agent and re-agent (the catalyst might be a third chemical, it might be heat – perhaps from placing the test tube over a Bunsen burner – or it may simply be the physical act of shaking the ingredients. In the *Bio*chemical reactions that take place within our bodies, *enzymes* [often vitamins] are typically the catalysts.) This universal concept can be seen in many other places as well, from the three basic components of the atom, to the Christian Trinity, to the three branches of government.

By applying this idea to the issue of disease-causation, a lot of troubling enigmas can be simplified: Why do some people get sick while others break all the rules and remain healthy? If tobacco is a carcinogen, why do some smokers not get cancer? Why do some people practically live on candy, saturated fat, and emotional negativity, and never get ill? Why do certain measures help one patient, yet fail with another? Why do some things come back, some never go away, and others just go away for good by themselves?

The answer is that *no one thing is ever responsible for any disease*. Rather, *three inter-reacting factors* are simultaneously necessary in every case:

1) There must be an *Active* force – that is, something detrimental must *act* on the body. This could be a germ, a poison, radiation, a physical injury, and so forth.

But these things are ceaselessly in contact with our bodies, and we do not all continually fall sick *en masse*. So there has to be more to it than just this. (Needless to say, one or another of these active agents might sometimes be *so overwhelming* that the other forces are rendered virtually irrelevant – a severe blow to the head, for instance, or a massive dose of lethal radiation. But this is the exception to the rule, not the general rule, and even in cases of massive poisoning or epidemic infections there is typically some small number of survivors, indicating that other factors are involved.)

2) There must be a *Receptive* force – that is, something in the body, sometimes referred to as the 'ground', must be already weakened or out-of-balance and thus *already receptive to being abnormally acted upon*. For instance, it might be a gut lining inflamed because of poor nutrition, a liver weakened by long-term drug or alcohol abuse, a congenitally weak heart, or any tissue that has been overwhelmed by the degenerative effects of long-term stress and tension.

4

But even if such an Active-to-Receptive intermingling occurs, and the body takes a turn toward illness, we have massive disease-controlling abilities: the immune system, the hormonal system, the nervous system, etc., should spring into action. So if our natural healing forces do not put a stop to this, there must still be *something else* going on.

3) There must be a *Conciliating* force – something inside us, against all of nature's best intentions, must inappropriately allow, or perhaps even encourage, the sickness to take hold and persist: more precisely, it must *fail* to *prevent* the body from *stopping* the active agent from damaging the receptive tissue. This 'something' is usually most perceptible as a malfunctioning **immune system**. And here is the key: as we shall see, the strength and viability of our immunity (and *all* our disease-fighting capabilities) is a joint function of physical, *emotional, psychological, and spiritual factors.*

This is why not all cigarette smokers get cancer. Tobacco *is* a carcinogen, but if a particular smoker was born with a "good constitution", if he or she eats well, exercises, and takes good care of the body in other ways, then he or she *may* luck out and not give the carcinogen enough weakened tissue to act upon. Or, if he or she has a really positive inner emotional and psychological life, then perhaps the immune system will simply not allow any cancerous activity to get out of control. (Despite these possibilities, I implore you not to risk it. Life is risky enough without cigarettes.)

Looked at from the opposite perspective, many people are warm, loving, even happy-go-lucky, and *do* get cancer. Some people jog and eat plenty of fresh vegetables and *do* get heart disease. Things are not as simple or linear as we might like them to be. It all comes down to matters of proportion and blending among three simultaneous causes, some within our control (e.g., diet, exercise, etc.), and some not in our control (e.g., genetics – though I reserve the right to partially revise this statement later on when we talk about *epi*genetics).

The particular pieces of the puzzle that comprise the three factors will differ in every individual case (a bacterium here, a virus there, a poor diet here, a poor attitude there). So while it is much too simplistic to say that there is One cause of illness, we *can* say:

There will always be an interwoven Triad of these three fundamental 'forces' behind any illness.

This 3-factor convergence is the "real" cause of pain and sickness.

The body is a whole, integrated, system. Everything is connected to everything. Since illness and pain are caused by an interaction of variable factors, it only makes sense that a single approach to all healing could not be sufficient. Rather than a limited *linear* way of thinking about health and disease as having only one cause (for instance, "germs") and only one appropriate response (for instance, "drugs"), we need to take a *holistic* approach that considers the entire set of circumstances.

2.   WHAT EXACTLY IS 'HOLISTIC HEALING', AND HOW CAN IT HELP ME?

In the old model, the body was looked at as a machine and the doctor as a mechanic: if something was wrong, fix it, or take it out and replace it. I prefer to look at the body as a garden and the doctor as a gardener: are these plants getting enough nutrients and water down to their roots, are these flowers getting enough sunlight?

Holistic healing, as the word implies, is about the *whole* situation. In other words, holistic healing must be concerned with *all* the many diverse aspects of life and health. This means that one therapy or practice, standing by itself, can never be considered "holistic" – chiropractic is not holistic if it assumes that spinal subluxations are the only cause of every pain or disease, acupuncture is not holistic if it insists that an imbalance in the flow of *ch'i* is the only cause of every illness. **To be holistic, *all three factors* discussed above must be considered and addressed.**

Also, no therapy can be described as holistic simply because it is "not western medicine." Western medicine has just as much a place in a holistic system as every other healing art. Of course, like every other healing art it is an integrated role, not an exclusive role. When seen in their proper light, the various treatment modalities are **not in competition** with each other. They are **not "instead of"** each other. They are *complementary*, they *supplement* each other: no healing art can do everything for everyone. "The whole range of healing systems that the genius of the human race has so patiently worked out,"[*] as Ted Kaptchuk once described them, are at their most effective, and are most helpful to *you*, when they work together cooperatively.

~

So turning now from the cause of illness to the process of healing, we can define 'Holistic Healing' in terms of the same three forces.

For a body to heal:

1) An *Active force for repair* of damaged tissue must be activated or added to the body. In other words, the body must start doing its job again. This may happen naturally with no outside help (perhaps just time), or it may be enhanced by outside help in the form of some kind of actively-stimulating healing remedy (a medicinal drug, an herbal remedy, etc.) or healing technique (a chiropractic or osteopathic adjustment, an acupuncture

---

[*] Ted Kaptchuk, *The Healing Arts,* Summit Books, NY, 1987 p. 48

7

treatment, a dental treatment, etc.), or something else that either artificially replaces a malfunctioning bodily process (typically the job of medical drugs or surgery, and often necessary in crises) or, better yet, *nudges the body itself back into appropriate action.* But this active 'nudge' is only one piece of the solution.

2) Meanwhile, the damaged, unbalanced tissue must now become *receptive to the healing action, receptive to the healing 'nudge'.* This is where basic good health habits and a healthy lifestyle come into play (nutrition, exercise, relaxation, regular massage, hatha yoga, hygiene, flossing, fasting, etc.), so that the tissues of the body no longer present an *obstacle* to healing but provide a healthy 'ground' where healing can easily take place. If our physical bodies are so badly cared for as to be unreceptive to healing, then no medicine, no technique, no remedy, and no amount of happiness are likely to help very much. Remember that your body is a sacred Temple and treat it well.

3) Finally, in order for the active healing forces in the body to be *capable* of repairing the damaged-but-now-receptive tissue, the overall psyche must be in a state in which the great tendency (consciously or not) is in the direction of life and health. The state of our **psyche** (mind, heart and spirit), through powerful interventions (see Chapter 5, below) in the endocrine, cardiovascular, nervous, and immune systems, provides this third healing force that either reconciles a poisonous substance and weak tissue to disease, or *reconciles a healing action and strong tissue to health.*

Again, even though the specific details will vary with each individual case, **an overall blueprint of this Triad of Healing** (and this all-embracing threefold blueprint is how I define 'Holistic') is present *in every case* – and each of the three forces may be affected in multiple ways

All three forces are critically necessary, but the third factor, in my opinion, is the most important consideration in healing, both because of the extraordinary potential power of our own mind and consciousness, and because it is often given such short shrift in our mechanistic culture.

3.   MY DOCTOR SAYS "IT'S ALL IN YOUR HEAD." IS IT?

I always find this notion – which many of my patients have had thrown in their faces by irritated practitioners who couldn't help them (and therefore reverted to **"blaming the victim"**) – extremely bizarre. And it is bizarre because it misunderstands reality on so many levels. Hidden within it lies the discredited notion that the physical body and the mind are completely distinct and separate entities (a notion long discredited by modern science). Within it lies the emotionally childish habit of blaming others – coupled with the arrogant assumption that the health care provider is *supposed* to be able to help absolutely everyone, and if he or she can't do so it must be the patient's fault (therefore, the doctor is off the hook). And within it lies a total misunderstanding of what the phenomenal power of the mind actually represents – this of course is borne of a *misguided absolute faith* in those same discredited canons of 19th century mechanical materialism.

Of course **it's in your head. Everything is!** There is nothing that *isn't* in your head. If you see some children playing in the yard, your experience of seeing them playing is occurring in your mind, i.e., in your head. If you feel pain in your knee, your experience of feeling pain is occurring in your mind. And for that matter, if you feel well again after taking some prescription drug, your experience of feeling well is only occurring in your mind. Nowhere else.

This is why I loved the Harry Potter books:

Harry: Is this all real? Or is it just happening inside my head?

Dumbledore: Of course it's happening inside your head Harry. Why should that mean that it's not real?

Not only is it *real*, but it is *empowering beyond measure.*
But it's not your "fault", and this kind of accusation is just a classic deflection tactic for practitioners who want to avoid responsibility, or 'friends' who have lost their patience and sympathy, and it just turns attention away from where it ought to be – *healing.*
On the other side of the same coin, we have all heard the words, spoken derisively, "Oh, that's just the placebo effect." We know that it is possible for someone to feel better, and for symptoms to go away, "merely because they mistakenly *believed* they were given real medicine".

9

"Just" the placebo effect? "Merely" because they believed? Hearing these sentiments never ceases to astonish me! I would submit that the placebo effect – *the ability of our consciousness to dramatically affect the physical world* – is arguably the most powerful force in the universe. It assures us that we have immense power to heal ourselves, without needing much or any help from medical doctors, chiropractors, herbalists, or anybody else. It is a force that, to be useful, would have to be harnessed, and that is certainly not easy: but if we *were* able to harness it, if we could learn to consciously and deliberately use this force at will, it is beyond anything that drug companies could ever come up with.

The ultimate conclusion to be drawn from the fact of the placebo effect is *not* that pain and illness are 'merely' or 'only' in our heads, or that we are easily fooled and our psychological weakness makes it 'our fault' (remember: *three* things are happening, and the state of your mind, with all its depth and complexity, is only one of them). **The placebo effect does not belittle us. It empowers us.** It tells us that we have profound possibilities, and that we can take charge of our own health. It promises that we need never underestimate our capacity to heal.

Consider the fantastic implications of the following information found in Dr. Bernie Siegel's book *Love, Medicine and Miracles,* in which the cardiologist discusses the results of studies of people with multiple personalities inhabiting one body:

> *"One personality may be a diabetic, while the other is not. Allergies and drug sensitivities may be present in one personality, but not in others. If one personality burns the body with a cigarette, the mark may disappear when the other personality is in control and reappear when the first personality reappears."*[*]

This, it seems to me, demonstrates that our self-healing potential is limitless! But *how can we deliberately harness* this incredible power?

It turns out that the body does not respond to logical words or direct verbal commands (e.g., "fix the pancreas", or "heal the liver"). **But the body *does* respond to *emotional feelings* and *vivid pictorial images*.** Thus, by working on our emotional well-being (and as an aside, I would place *faith* and *prayer* within the Heart, not as intellectual activities), and through the conscious use of our Imagination (for example, by using guided visualization techniques) we can learn to send healing instructions into our body.

---

[*] Siegel, Bernie, *Love, Medicine and Miracles,* Harper and Row, NY, 1986, p.124

We'll talk more about emotional work soon. But here I want to say something about the power of your imagination. In Michael Gelb's book *Body Learning: An Introduction to the Alexander Technique*, he relates the story of an imagery experiment conducted by psychologist Alan Richardson. In this experiment, a group of young basketball players was divided into two groups. The first group was told to practice shooting baskets for an hour each day over a period of several weeks. The second group was told to stay off the court for these several weeks, but to spend an hour each day *imagining* that they were successfully shooting baskets, mentally going through all the motions and watching in their mind's eye as ball after ball left their fingertips and soared through the hoop. At the end of the experiment a competition was held. Everyone had improved, and those who had practiced only in their imagination performed as well as those who had actually practiced on the court: in fact, their muscle control, hand-eye coordination, aim, and overall skill had all improved by simply imagining the improvement.

~

We develop illnesses, in the words of Carl Simonton and Stephanie-Matthews-Simonton, "for honorable reasons".* In other words, **illness means that somewhere along the line our legitimate needs are not being met**: these needs may be physical, sexual, emotional, psychological, social, or spiritual. The Simontons learned long ago that **if we are not meeting our serious needs appropriately, we may have to meet them artificially through pain or illness.** (John Sarno found much success with many back-pain patients by simply getting them to *understand and accept* that their pain was being caused by tension, and there was really no physical, incurable, damage to their spine. This allowed their **fear** to subside, and be replaced with knowledge. Fear is a powerful "third force" in the triad of illness: negative attitudes of hopelessness and despondency can artificially and unnecessarily cause some people to give up the fight and spiral into sickness and death, only because *fear has convinced them that they have to.* Don't let yourself be hypnotized by something negative or hopeless someone else tells you.)

The realization that we have legitimate needs, that we are connected by a sacred system of give-and-take with other people and the world, is a liberating experience. It means that we have the right and the obligation to ask. It means that we have the right and the obligation to receive. It

---

* Carl O. Simonton, Stephanie Matthews-Simonton, *Getting Well Again,* Bantam Books, NY, 1984, p. 176

means that we have the right and the obligation to give. The recognition that one has contributed to one's ill health (which is true to one extent or another for *every* person and *every* case of illness) has nothing whatsoever to do with accepting guilt or blame. This would totally miss the point. **The real point is that we do have power, and our illnesses occur for respectable reasons.** The same internal forces that allowed disease to take hold in the first place can potentially be turned around and used for self-healing. There is immense power in this.

In fact, there is really no such thing as powerlessness: it is just a question of whether our power works against us by default, or for us by conscious intent.

So the next time someone says "it's all in your head", rise up to your full stature and say, *"you're damn right."* Then find someone with more class to hang out with.

4.   I CAN'T FIX PROBLEMS CAUSED BY MY GENES AND DNA, CAN I?

Unless you left college very recently, you have been taught that the DNA in our genes determines our anatomical characteristics and our physiological processes, and their decisions are absolute and unchangeable – as a result, if we happen to be prone to certain illnesses or physical complaints, or are otherwise dissatisfied with our physical makeup, it is simply too bad: we are victims of our genes.

But it turns out we are *not* victims of our genes, except in the rarest of cases. Only about 2% of the population suffer from those devastating problems that are inexorably caused by a defective or missing gene: aside from possible symptomatic relief, it is sadly true that little can be done about this (though hopefully some wonderful future research will find a way to alter the chromosomal structure or lead to some other form of real relief).

For most of us, however, the conventional belief that our genetic makeup determines our fate, turns out to be not-so-true after all. Recent discoveries in **Epigenetics**, a new branch of biology that studies how environmental signals are translated into gene expression, have changed all that.

The first thing that was found is that around each strand of DNA there is a *'protein sleeve.'* This sleeve serves as a barrier between the information contained in the DNA strand and the rest of the cell's environment. DNA provides a blueprint for how new proteins are to be formed (most of our physical structure – our muscles, organs, etc. – as well as most of the enzymes that determine how internal chemical processes will proceed – are made of protein). But in order for the blueprint in the DNA to be 'read' so that the protein can be made, *the sleeve around that piece of DNA has to be unwrapped* so that the information is available. Otherwise, it cannot be acted upon and the blueprint in the DNA remains dormant.

So what has to happen is that some kind of 'signal' must arrive at the protein sleeve to 'tell' it that a piece of the DNA it is covering is needed and it has to unravel at that spot. Once this happens, the code is recognized by other cellular elements and the particular protein molecule is assembled: this is what biologists mean when they say that a gene is "expressed".

Two important questions arise: (1) what kind of 'signals' cause the protein sleeve to unravel and allow the gene's message to be read and acted upon ("expressed"), and (2) is that gene's information "written in stone", as we say, so that nothing can ever be done to alter it and we are at its mercy?

Let's assume for the moment that all 'signals' are in fact chemicals that get into the cells. The proteins comprising the 'sleeve' have receptors that recognize particular chemicals as signals that, when touched, spur them to open up. It is easy enough to imagine that if a particular protein is lacking somewhere, this could cause a chemical to enter the cell and slide over to that part of sleeve surrounding the required DNA and cause it to open up and make some of that protein.

But this simple statement actually reveals something extremely important: **Our genetic activity is *not determined by the genes themselves!* On the contrary, our genetic activity is determined by *chemical influences in the cell's environment*** that cross the membrane into the cell. **In other words, it is the *environment* that causes our 'fate'**, not our DNA. And yes, we *can* affect our cells' environment in many, many ways (what foods we eat being just one such way). This is why I reserved the right to alter my previous statement that our genes are beyond our control. We are *not* 'helpless victims' of our genes.

For instance, suppose you have a gene that, if expressed, causes you to develop diabetes. If the protein sleeve around that gene is never unwrapped, the gene can cause no harm! Sure enough, epigenetic researchers have found that the protein sleeve can be affected by a good diet and an active lifestyle: these behaviors cause *different chemical signals* to enter the cell than if you ate poorly and had a generally unhealthy lifestyle. In fact, a healthy lifestyle can actually *tighten* the sleeve.

But there's more! Not only could this protect *you* from diabetes despite having this gene, but the *tighter protein sleeve gets passed down through heredity* along with the underlying gene. In other words, **our lifestyle choices not only affect *our* health, but they can affect *future generations as well.*** If this information doesn't make your eyes widen and start to water, I don't know what will. (And if you know something about biochemist Rupert Sheldrake's **'morphic resonance'** work – demonstrating that *memory is inherent and pervasive in Nature* – you see that the healing and preventive possibilities are even *more* profound.)

It is not just food and exercise that change the cell's environment and affect our genetic expression. The fate of our cells is controlled by the chemicals in the blood, but the chemicals in our blood are modified and attuned by the way we perceive our life. In other words, our thoughts, emotions, and beliefs, affect our cells as well.

5.   *HOW* DO MY *EMOTIONS* AFFECT MY *PHYSICAL* PAIN OR SICKNESS?

Consider this: In the center of our brain is an area called the *hypothalamus*. Researchers have long known that the various sections of the hypothalamus are concerned with such things as pleasure, pain, sexuality, hunger, and all our emotions. Just above the hypothalamus are the two enormous **cerebral hemispheres**, the seat of our higher thinking functions. Thousands of nerves connect the hypothalamus with the cerebral hemispheres, which means that information about our thoughts and emotions are continually being exchanged.

The hypothalamus borders an open chamber called the third ventricle, which is filled with cerebrospinal fluid (a moving fluid that cushions, bathes, and nourishes the cells of the brain and spinal cord). Also bordering the third ventricle are the *pineal gland* and the *pituitary gland.*

The pineal gland (which some esoteric traditions believe is a physical manifestation of a '**third eye**', the 'eye of the soul' – and it does in fact have anatomical similarities to our eyes) releases melatonin, which regulates sleep and may affect the immune system and have anti-aging effects, into the cerebrospinal fluid. But the pineal gland is *also* probably the source for another fascinating chemical, **DMT** (Dimethyltryptamine), that is likewise found in the cerebrospinal fluid. DMT is also widespread in the plant kingdom *in plants that are commonly used in shamanic rituals*. It can produce powerful near-death and mystical experiences, and is hypothesized to be released at birth, death, and during vivid dreams. It has been called "the spirit molecule".

The pituitary gland is called 'the master gland'. This is because it tells the other glands of the hormonal system what to do: i.e., by sending out its own chemical signals into the bloodstream it tells the thyroid gland when to speed up the body's metabolism by producing more thyroid hormone, or it tells the adrenals when to cut down the production of cortisol, etc. Of course, it makes these decisions after receiving chemical signals *from* the various glands as well as messages from the hypothalamus. The pituitary is thus like a Master Conductor, listening to all the instruments and conducting the body's great chemical symphony.

But the hypothalamus *composed* the symphony, and is constantly at work updating and re-writing parts of it and *sending new instructions to the conductor*. It is inspired to create these new compositions in response to neural communication between higher thinking centers and its own emotional content, as well as the spiritual messages it receives from the pineal gland through chemical messages in the cerebrospinal fluid, and with continual feedback from the pituitary gland, which, in turn, is in constant contact with the endocrine glands throughout the body (which, according to some spiritual traditions, are the physical representatives of the chakras – which links them to the movement of *ch'i* through the invisible acupuncture meridians, and the possible arousal of kundalini).

*In other words, this constant communication amongst physical, emotional, intellectual and spiritual aspects of our being, causes chemical changes within the cerebrospinal fluid (which bathes the entire brain and central nervous system, exchanging information at all times), as well as all the powerful yet delicate hormones that are released by the endocrine glands – which enter the bloodstream and **then go on to enter and affect every single cell in the body** (in some ways that we understand, but undoubtedly also in myriad ways we have yet to discover.)*

So here we see *some* of **the extraordinary links between mind, heart, body, and spirit,** demonstrating how we end up with *physical results of our thoughts, emotions and beliefs*: these physical results change the very content of our blood, they bathe and communicate with the brain, and they enter and affect the environment of every one of the trillions of cells in our bodies. Add to this the new research about DNA and how by changing the cell's environment we can change our genetic expression, and we see a hint, at the very least, of the immense potential to heal ourselves and determine our own fate that always lies within us.

We may not yet know all the exact mechanisms for this enormous healing potential, but I can assure you even now that if you choose to experience a world full of love and kindness, your body will respond in many healthy ways. If you choose to experience a world of fear and hatred, your overall health will be compromised. This cannot be 'measured' in a laboratory. That does not change the fact that it is true. Every emotion changes the fabric of the body.

~

And this discussion of hormones brings us back to the subject of *stress* and how it affects our health.

We know that stress causes a specific variety of responses in the body. We know that these physiological responses are healthy and valuable in moments of danger. But under *chronic* stress, when these physiological actions continue unabated because the stressful danger never seems to end, the mind and body can be badly damaged.

16

When we perceive love and joy in our lives, the body releases chemicals like oxytocin, dopamine, and serotonin into the bloodstream. These chemicals promote vitality and health. But when the hypothalamus recognizes danger (it may be a saber-tooth tiger, or it may be an angry boss, a sour relationship, financial hardship, a fear of crime or terrorism, etc.), it tells the pituitary to order the adrenal glands to secrete protective *stress hormones* (e.g., adrenaline and cortisol) into the bloodstream. These hormones do three particular things:

> (1) they **contract blood vessels in the *gut***, so that during the crisis energy is not wasted on digestion, and more blood is instead sent into the muscles of the arms and legs which may be called upon to run or fight;

> (2) they **suppress the *immune system***, and the ability to inhibit or shut down inflammatory responses, again so that energy is not wasted (we can fight off the flu virus *after* we have escaped the tiger); and

> (3) they **contract blood vessels in the *fore*brain** (which relates to the *conscious* mind and our ability to think things through), and send the blood back to the *hind*brain (which relates to the *subconscious* mind that runs our reflex activity): after all, this is no time for thinking, this is the time for acting!

This is all well and good in moments of danger. But if the source of stress continues and continues, if we are besieged by unresolved problems and worries, or if we are overwhelmed by unresolved fears that continue to stress us out even if the external cause has disappeared (PTSD is an extreme example of this, but it does not have to be that extreme to be a serious problem), then notice what happens:

(1) *our digestive system functions poorly*, which can lead to a myriad of issues involving pain, malabsorption of nutrients that our cells need to maintain health and life, bowel issues, etc.

(2) *lowered immunity* opens us up to attacks from bacteria, viruses, and other pathogens that should have been stopped, and allows inflammation to get out of control (evidence is rapidly accruing in research circles that a vast number of illnesses are connected to **chronic inflammation**: diabetes, heart disease, stroke, Alzheimer's, cancer, obesity, allergies,

Parkinson's, colitis, Crohn's disease, asthma, psoriasis, neurological problems, lethargy and fatigue, migraines, and various other illnesses[*]).

(3) we become *less able to think clearly* (some studies suggest that the inhibition of neurons by stress hormones may be a root cause of **depression**).

The obvious need to break these cycles of chronic stress is why **relaxation** (to calm the freneticisms of the body) and **meditation** (to calm the freneticisms of the mind) are critical requirements for healing.

A body filled with **tension** will suffer from fatigue, stiffness and pain. It may be clumsy and unattractive. It may be cut off from sensations of pain (which provide important warnings) as well as from feelings of

---

[*] You can see why it is so very important that **inflammation** be stopped and/or prevented. Here's a useful general protocol to help do so: **1**. *Eat a Low Glycemic Diet* – filled with green leafy vegetables, avocadoes, nuts and legumes, seeds, cruciferous vegetables (broccoli, cauliflower, kale, cabbage, Brussels sprouts), as well as vegetables, fruits and berries that come in a wide variety of colors. But do not drink commercial fruit juices. Drink water! **2**. *Avoid (at least), or Eliminate (at best): all sugar and sweeteners*, all white flour products (breads, cereals and pasta), white rice, white potatoes and other nightshades if you think you are sensitive to them, all 'junk food', all dairy foods, all packaged and/or processed 'foods', grains (they can all contribute to inflammation, but if you cannot eliminate them all for a period of time, at least eliminate grains containing gluten: wheat, rye, spelt, couscous, barley, bulgur, and any foods that contain these. Stick to small amounts of brown rice, quinoa, buckwheat). **3**. *Eat small, frequent, meals*. Eat *Mindfully*). **4**. *Use Turmeric and Ginger*, but otherwise do *not* eat more-than-*mildly*-spicy foods. **5**. Eat *naturally fermented foods like sauerkraut.* **6**. *Use oils sparingly* (a little coconut oil for cooking, a small amount of extra virgin olive oil on a salad – lemon juice is better – do not use safflower oil, corn oil, peanut oil, canola oil, or 'vegetable' oil. Don't *cook* with olive oil.) **7**. *Avoid commonly suspected allergens*: corn, soy, alcohol, caffeine, yeast, dairy, eggs, sugar, peanuts, tobacco, and any foods you know or suspect give you problems. **8**. *Get exercise every day.* **9**. If you have trouble sleeping *at least six hours per night*, explore remedies. **10**. *Relax and Meditate every day.* **11**. Do something each day that *makes you feel happy and useful*, and *appreciate other people* who do the same. **12**. Try to *rid your home of dangerous chemicals*, mold, heavy metals, pollutants **13**. Consider taking some of these *supplements*: **(a)** Vitamins C, B-complex, E (no more than 200 IU per day), D3, K; **(b)** Flaxseed Oil or Fish Oil, 2-4 g/day (certified free of pesticides and heavy metals), **(c)** Pancreatic (Digestive) Enzymes, **(d)** a Hydrochloric Acid supplement for the GI tract, **(e)** Selenium, **(f)** CoQ10, **(g)** Folic Acid (best in folate form), **(h)** L-Glutamine, and **(i)** *definitely take Probiotics.*

18

pleasure. Chronic tension will impede the free circulation of blood, nerve energy, and *ch'i,* causing the body to deteriorate and age more quickly, and it will have difficulty recognizing or 'hearing' important signals coming from the internal or external environment. Fortunately, there are countless excellent techniques of 'body work' (e.g., massage, tai chi, Feldenkrais, etc.), that help teach overexcited westerners *how to relax.*

Relaxation does not mean sitting around being lazy. Slouching in front of the TV with a pile of chips, or even lying happily on the beach, does not mean that one is relaxed. All sorts of muscles can be tight and tense while we are doing these things. Relaxation *means only using those muscles that are necessary for what we are doing in a given moment,* be it sitting on the couch watching TV or carrying a box of books up a flight of stairs. In other words, we can relax and be active at the same time: in fact, if we can learn to do this, then productive, efficient, relaxed work can *increase* our energy, rather than making us tired.

People who practice regular **meditation** routinely discover not only that their health improves, but that all aspects of their lives are affected in beneficial ways. The deepest purpose of meditation is to silence the endless blather of the chattering "monkey mind" so that, in the stillness and silence that follows, a higher divine force can arise in our being and lift our consciousness up into higher spiritual realities. But meditation is also, to be sure, a useful tool for physical healing: it lowers the amount of stress hormones released into the bloodstream, it causes brain-wave patterns to show less excitability (which changes attitudes and moods), and all of this lowers the risk of heart attacks and strokes and cancer, among many other ailments.

I also recommend **hypnosis** as an excellent tool for shifting our consciousness away from negative thinking, self-destructive behaviors, limiting beliefs, paralyzing negative emotions, and other stressful psychological blockages to healing and growth.

Of course, the *best* way to reduce stress, and ***the most powerful healing force of all,*** is not a secret. So let me conclude this chapter on emotions and healing with another great quote from Bernie Siegel, M.D.

> **I am convinced that *unconditional love* is the most powerful known stimulant of the immune system. If I told patients to raise their blood levels of immune globulins or killer T cells, no one would know how. But if I can teach them to love themselves and others fully, the same changes occur automatically. The truth is: Love heals.**[*]

---

[*] Siegel, Bernie, *Love, Medicine & Miracles,* Harper & Row, NY, 1986, p.181

6. WHAT IS 'ENERGY HEALING'? IS IT REAL? CAN IT HELP ME?

Energy healing is grounded in the very ancient contention, verified by contemporary science, that there is a flow of energy within and surrounding the body: an invisible, permeating, energy '**field**' within which the material body is immersed. This energy field extends outwards for up to 15 feet and operates primarily at frequencies matching those of the earth's electromagnetic field. It is assumed by most energy healers that this energetic field is *primary*, meaning that it serves as a kind of underlying 'template' for the body which forms, exists, and grows within it (rather than the reverse idea that the physical body is primary, and the field is created secondarily as an effect of matter. But a bit of *matter*, as quantum physics has revealed, is really just a region in space where 'the field is extremely intense'. **Einstein, for example, noted that "the field is the only reality."**) The field vibrates, or, perhaps more accurately, the field *is* vibration: higher and lower frequencies of vibration are reflections, and perhaps causes, of our state of well-being. Lastly, it is assumed by energy healers that any hindrance or disruption to the free and natural movement of energy throughout this living field can affect the body adversely and initiate illness or pain, but by working with the field itself (i.e., by removing 'blockages' to the flow of energy, calming places of excess energy, and/or increasing energy where it has decreased) such illnesses may be improved, healed, or prevented.

Consciousness, vibration, and intuition, are all interconnected; probably just different ways of viewing the same phenomena. If our thoughts and feelings delve into negativity, our vibrational frequency slows down, and our awareness and perception close down. If we raise our level of vibration, we become more conscious, we feel more alive, we are connected once again with our own body and all the people and nature around us. This means that raising any piece of this continuum raises all of it (of course, the reverse is also true).

Our emotional state can clue us in, at all times, to what our vibrational state is like. So the simplest way to raise your vibrations, increase your consciousness, and increase your intuition, is to do things or think about things that make you feel good - happy, positive, hopeful, grateful, etc. (If you do not like to think in terms of concepts such as vibration, intuition, or even consciousness, just recall that **the body's** *chemistry* – **hormones, neurotransmitters, enzymes, etc., – is all affected by the state of our emotions** whether we "believe" in such things or not.)

Here are some specific ways to raise the vibrational level of the energy field: Meditate, relax, stretch, play a sport or game you enjoy, listen to music, play music, paint, sculpt, draw, watch a Marx Brothers film, play with a pet, listen to children's laughter, watch an inspiring movie, read an inspiring book, exercise (something you enjoy), hug, pray, take long slow deep breaths, make a list of people or things you are grateful for, walk through a forest, sit by a lake or ocean (or jump right in), or take a bath or shower, or *just go do something nice for someone.*

What is an energy blockage? What does it do?

This can be compared, somewhat simplistically but nonetheless accurately, to water flowing through a hose as it waters a garden. If there is a blockage in the hose, there will be less water beyond the blockage, and there will be a pressure buildup (and possibly a leak or overflow of water) behind the blockage. Either way, it is easy to see how too little water or too much water can lead to problems for the garden.

In the case of subtle energies flowing through channels in the energy field, a lessening of energy in one place would most likely result in weakness, fatigue, or some kind of symptom (physical or psychological) due to **loss of vitality**, while a high-pressured back-up of energy could lead to a symptom reflecting the **overstimulation** of a corresponding body part or some emotional aspect of your life: intense, backed-up energetic pressures might lead to emotional tension or anxiety, or could lead to a build-up in the physical body of heat and **inflammation** (which, more and more is being recognized as a critical contributor to a whole assortment of contemporary illnesses.)

What *causes* blockages and imbalances in energy flow?

Generally, the same things that we see in physical illness and injury: it could be poisons and toxins; bacteria or other pathogens; physical trauma; poor nutrition; a sedentary lifestyle; negativity, stress and emotional trauma; even hereditary problems. But it is important to note that, on the one hand, blockages and imbalances in the body's energy field often arise long *before* physical symptoms appear (a fact that empowers us with possibilities of prevention), and they often remain, to one degree or another, *long after* such symptoms have been resolved by physical means (which is why many recurrences and relapses are really not so mysterious after all).

It is also worth noting that many imbalances in our body's subtle energy field can be due to subtle, intangible, causes – i.e., causes that orthodox medicine is generally unaware of or uninterested in: negative emotions; fear; pent-up rage; the unconscious results of forgotten emotional trauma; karmic effects or even obscure cosmic events; or perhaps the effects of coming into contact with, and resonating with, the imbalanced energy fields of others. For instance, some people are extremely sensitive to all sorts of conflict and emotion taking place in their surroundings, or even in the world at large, and all of us are undoubtedly more sensitive to these things than we may realize or admit.

I hasten to add that most experienced medical professionals are certainly intuitively aware that something more than mechanical material science is involved in healing, even if we cannot articulate in ordinary language what this 'something' is, and even if it cannot be studied in a test tube. In any event, the healing of the physical body and the healing of the energy body are not separate and should be treated holistically as one.

It's probably impossible not to. Nevertheless, if you are focusing all your attention solely on the physical elements of your life, and you find that efforts to grow and change are not bearing much fruit, or you keep coming back to the same unwanted place, or the same problems recur over and over again, you might want to consider that you are only working on *one half of your total reality* and your energy body needs attention.

How can blockages be removed? How can the free and healthful movement of subtle energies be enhanced?

Generally speaking, in the same ways that we can raise our overall vibrational level; although it may be useful to also focus your **attention** (since energy follows thought), and perhaps place your **hands**, on areas where you think blockages may exist (where you feel a symptom, where you feel pain or discomfort or muscle tightness, or wherever your intuition leads you). The list of suggestions bears repeating, with some added variations: relaxation, meditation, chanting, listening to music that relaxes you or simply makes you smile, smiling itself (even if for no apparent reason), drawing your attention into the body and focusing on places of pain or discomfort while trying to gently "let the pain go", deep breathing, movement and physical exercise, yoga, tai chi, chi gung, dancing, laughing, crying, hugging, praying, doing fun and creative arts that you enjoy, having sex (in a loving, giving way, never in a demanding or selfish way), observing your negative emotions without judgment (being sure to remember that we all have them, we are all in the same boat) and learning to accept and love yourself, taking time each day to simply feel happy and grateful, playing with a child, playing with a pet, or even just taking a walk through the woods – breathing the fresh air, smelling the flowers, listening to the birds and the wind, or perhaps contemplating the stars.

One very powerful way to open up one's energy flow is to *forgive*. We don't forgive evil *acts*: we forgive another person their *weaknesses* – if for no other reason than because we recognize, deep down, that we *all* have weaknesses: in fact, we all have pretty much the *same* weaknesses ("there but for the Grace of God...."). In other words, forgiveness is really about oneself, recognizing the damage that our feelings of blame and resentment do to *us* and *choosing peace instead*. **Nothing stifles our life-affirming energies, and holds us down and binds us to a life of mediocrity, joylessness, sickness and pain, more completely than our unresolved feelings of indignation, anger, hatred and resentment that we cling to so determinedly**. Instead, we can accept that we are really all the same, we can choose not to be victims or accusers, we can cultivate compassion and forgiveness *for others and ourselves*. (A thousand years from now, what will it matter? A thousand light years from here, who really cares? *Breathe, smile, let it go*.)

Another powerful means for pushing through blockages and raising our vibrations, is to remember that life only lasts a short while, and to try and make every moment count passionately. When a bad mood, or overwhelming feelings of negativity, start to descend, try to remember that you could die in the next moment, or the person you are talking to, or ignoring, or even just thinking about, could die in the next moment, *and there may never be another chance to fill your lungs with the vibrancy and magnificence of life, there may never be another chance to say something kind, helpful, friendly or loving.* Each moment is precious. *This moment* is all we can ever be assured of. Why waste it on a bad mood?

It is also worthwhile to **find some time each day to be aware** of the energy fields that surround you and permeate you, and that surround and permeate everyone and every living thing: even if you don't see or feel these things, even if it all seems like a lot of silly hocus-pocus to your rational mind – in which case, just remember that science is well aware that every living cell exists within an electro-magnetic field and even gives off photons of light, so use the power of your imagination to imagine, "play pretend", and maybe get a little taste of these things.

I must add that all of these actions will work infinitely better and be infinitely more effective if you try to be awake, conscious, and self-attentive, while you are doing them. In other words, when you walk through the forest breathing in all the scents and sounds, wake yourself up and notice that *you* are walking through the forest, notice that *you* are experiencing the sights and sounds and scents, **notice** that *you* are **present**, and *feel your presence*.

Really feel it. In other words, don't allow life to only take place *outside you*, don't let your life pass you by unnoticed! *Experience your experiences consciously*. When you are hugging a friend, when you are playing with a child, when you are making love, wake yourself up, remember your presence, take a stop and take a breath, and really look into their eyes while simultaneously looking into your own soul, and *be present*. Feel *their* presence, and feel *your own* presence. (Presence isn't "a deeper awareness of what's going on around you." Presence is in awakening and inner conscious union with that sacred 'hidden' spark within you, that deep lovely vibration that is the most 'real' YOU.)

In fact, as you go through the days and months and years of your life, whenever you can remember this, *take a stop, feel what it feels like to be immersed in your body, observe what is happening around you, try to feel the* **connection** *between your body and the environment, and look deep within your heart and say "Here, and Now, I AM"*.

The vibrational fields that permeate and surround each cell, each body part, every person, and every life form, all merge and interweave and resonate with one another. Thus, an individual's energy field doesn't really come to an 'end' fifteen feet from the body. We now know that 'particles of matter' are really just miniature energy fields themselves, i.e., *tiny energy vortices*. Matter **appears** to be 'discrete': that is, a body **appears** to have finite boundaries that separate it from its environment. *Energy*, however, **does not have boundaries**; waves of energy extend *infinitely* through space. So, from the standpoint of the 'energy body', the spiritual principle that "**Everything is One**" is not a mystery – it's just an awareness of the infinite continuum of vibration and life.

When you turn inward and truly experience your own presence, far from being *isolated* you are more *deeply connected* to everyone and everything, for your inner sacred *presence* is eternally in a state of resonance with the great *Presence* of the entire living universe.

This great Oneness of Life takes place with or without our conscious awareness or participation. But why would we want to sleep through this marvelous show? Why would we want to contract and hide from reality?

25

To consider the body this way (that is, to acknowledge that we are more than just a conglomeration of mechanical atoms, that we are imbued with, and surrounded by, and in fact *are*, an energy field that connects us vibrationally with each other and with all of life), allows us to more deeply appreciate the exquisite wisdom of the body, and beyond that to appreciate the phenomenal wisdom of Nature, the wonder of healing, and the miracle of life itself, including our individual and mutual existence here on this third planet encircling a star called Sol in this far distant corner of a nondescript galaxy..

What does an 'Energy Healer' do?

So the key to energy healing is to open blockages, clear channels and pathways, and keep the energies of life moving freely and naturally, thus keeping the physical body and the energy body in a balanced, harmonious, alignment – all of which helps to prevent many problems, and allows and encourages the body to *heal* any problems that have already occurred, and then to *remain* healthy and strong. Like all healing, this is mostly up to the patient: an energy healer, like *any* healing practitioner, can ***only help***.

An energy healer may use many different 'techniques' to provide this help. I would suggest that the most important ones are psychological, and of these the most important is **intent**. When dealing with subtle energies, the *intention to help*, the *intention to be of service*, and the *intention (and willingness) to get out of the way* and allow oneself to be a conduit for higher forces (that one need not even understand), is, in my opinion, paramount. Along with this, the 'techniques' of clearing one's mind of negativity, opening one's heart to the patient, and being completely *present*, can open the energy healer's **intuition** to deeper levels so that he or she can receive guidance. But perhaps even more important than any of this, is making an internal effort to **drop the ego** and recognize that *"I am not doing anything* – whatever healing may occur is between the patient and higher sacred forces that I simply invite to use me." Offering **unconditional love**, of course, is always of benefit: vibrations *always* raise (or lower) other vibrations that they meet.

Beyond that, I would only say that an energy healer may make use of movement, breathing, touch, hand motions, acupuncture needles, biofeedback, neurofeedback, hypnosis, muscle testing, homeopathic remedies, prayer, flower essences, sound, music, crystals, pendulums, Rife frequencies, Bemer mats (electromagnetic therapy), light, candles, magnets, incense, massage, Reiki, aromatic oils, infrared light, vibration, chanting, or other means to help open channels, balance energies, and raise vibrations. Some practitioners even do healings over long distances, since, as noted, the life-energy continuum exists everywhere at once.

Some practitioners speak of clearing auras, some speak of opening chakras, some speak of running meridians, etc. Why do different energy healers describe what they do in so many ways?

One way to answer this, is to recognize that contemporary science has taught us that we can only *perceive* what we can *conceive* – in other words, Einstein and others came to realize that when scientists (or any of us) look into the world *we can only see what our prior concepts, beliefs, and thoughts, allow us to see*: "It is the theory," he said, "which decides what we can observe."* So a healer trained in a certain tradition will naturally see things according to the teachings of that tradition.

The energy field that surrounds and permeates a human body, or any living thing, is a complex of *many* fields – some that scientists know a good deal about (electromagnetic fields, brain and heart waves, light photons, infrared emission, etc.), and some that science as yet knows little or nothing about. It may be that the different energetic patterns (chakras, auras, etc.) that energy healers experience are different-but-interrelated *layers* of the total interwoven vibrational field that surrounds and permeates a body: again, different practitioners will work with different layers, different aspects, according to their training, experience, and intuitive abilities.

~

Energy healing may well be *the best preventive modality*. Once an illness or injury is present in the body, however, other *physical* treatment modalities (including drugs and surgery, which most definitely can be a godsend at times) may certainly be helpful or necessary. Nonetheless, energy balancing work is always a valuable *adjunct* in all cases, *during* the physical healing process as well as *after*.

Energy moves much faster than chemicals: ultimately, medical science will recognize that working with the body's energy is a more effective, lasting, and efficient way of healing than working only with slow-moving chemicals.

---

* Quoted in Malin, Prof. Shimon, *Nature Loves to Hide*, Oxford University Press, Oxford, UK, 2001, p. 31-32.

In fact, since most of our problems, whether physical or psychological, begin to crystalize in the energy body first, our non-physical reality should never be ignored.

A Final Word:

The most powerful healer is *You*.

As we have seen, the universe is nothing other than energy and vibration. But there is something else to note: The universe is 'homeopathic'. That is, 'like vibrations' seek and are drawn to 'like vibrations' – and as we also have seen, our vibrations reflect our emotional state.

What this means is, if you make an effort to *feel good* – to see the positive, to think and feel loving thoughts, to remember and appreciate the blessings you already have, to relax and allow yourself to feel content and happy, to remember the sacred center that is You and that is in Communion with the Divine and with all Beings, if you *let yourself feel happy and make a conscious effort to 'see' yourself healthy and strong and loved and well,* you will be sending healing vibrations into the world and more and more healing vibrations will come to you in an avalanche of abundance simply by virtue of sweeping the negativity out of their way. This is not about 'lying'. It is about telling the universe and God the Truth about what you truly want, and showing gratitude for it (this is key) *even now.* The universe is 'Response to Request' – and for the Universe, there is no condition that cannot be improved.

Maybe you are searching among the branches,
for what only appears in the roots.

- *Rumi*

7. WHO ARE *YOU* AND HOW CAN *YOU* HELP ME?
(aka 'ABOUT THE AUTHOR')

I received my Doctor of Chiropractic degree in 1981, and began practicing in the East Village in NYC. Now, many years and many adventures later (I've also been a math and physics teacher and briefly practiced law in Boston and the Berkshires), I find myself in Upstate New York. My practice has evolved greatly since my East Village days, and I now have a very unique and eclectic practice – and I love it!

I would love to see *you* for regular holistic treatments. I can assure you that you will feel safe, listened to, cared about, and respected. I'm at 53 Rock City Road, Woodstock, NY 12498. (Contact (845) 750-9652 or Andrew @AndrewCort.com.)

WHAT I DO:

I spend a full 90 minutes on each patient visit. I work from toe to head and beyond. Throughout each session I devote attention to **relaxation**, **energy balancing**, and the near-magical effects of gentle, heart-felt, **human touch**. A typical session begins with responding to your specific pain or complaint, if any (often using tools from **Applied Kinesiology**, **nutrition**, and **muscle release work**, but this always depends). I then begin working at the feet with the patient on their back, using a combination of foot massage, foot alignment, and **reflexology**. Next, I may do some **visceral manipulation** if called for, and I often work on the all-important **core hip flexors and diaphragm**. Next I have you turn over on your stomach, and I do a **full spine alignment** (*no crunching, no cracking, all very gentle* – that's all it takes when you are deeply relaxed), and probably a good bit of leg, back, and shoulder **massage**: I may use a hand-held **infrared, cold laser,** or **vibrating** massager to relax muscles and stimulate healing. I then have you turn over again; I sit at the head of the table and do some **craniosacral balancing** work. Finally, I have you close your eyes and I take you on a **guided visualization** journey to bring you even deeper into relaxation and stimulate your self-healing abilities through the power of your imagination. The visualization always ends with a focus on your **heart**, and letting positive, happy, memories and emotions soak into the cells of your body.

FEES: My current fee is $85 per session. I do not deal with insurance companies, but *no one is ever turned away for financial reasons*. I do

29

not work for the insurance companies: I work for you. I am happy to accept *whatever you can comfortably and fairly afford*.

***

Thank you for reading this pamphlet – ***knowledge enhances healing***.

PS. If you enjoyed this pamphlet, you might appreciate some of my many books, including:

The Beauty and Nobility of Life: *The Restoration of Meaning in a World Overwhelmed by Commercialism, Scientism, & Fundamentalism* [*** Winner of the **2017 1ˢᵗ Place Gold Award** from *Nautilus Book Awards*, in the category "USA Spiritual Growth and Development".]

Eat Healthy: *Live Longer, Live Kinder*

The Sacred Chalice – Women in the Bible: *The Psychological and Spiritual Meaning of Their Stories*

Our Healing Birthright: *Taking Responsibility for Ourselves and Our Planet*

The Door is Open: *The 7 Steps of Spiritual Awakening that Western Scripture and Mythology Have Been Trying to Tell Us All Along*

Symbols, Meaning, and the Sacred Quest: *Spiritual Awakening in Jewish, Christian, and Islamic Stories*

Love, Wisdom, and God: *The Longing of the Western Soul*

***

Please Note: I am available for Talks and Seminars on these and related topics.

-    *Andrew Cort*
www.AndrewCort.com

May we have peace on Earth,
goodwill toward all men, women, and especially children,
and all that lives and breathes

Made in the USA
Columbia, SC
13 October 2018